ESSENTIAL OILS

ENJOY THE BENEFITS OF HOMEMADE ESSENTIAL OILS RECIPES FOR HEALING, BEAUTY CARE NAD RELAXING THERAPY

Table of Contents

Introduction

When you're like me, you have a palatable stash of prevalent oils and are constantly looking for approaches to utilize them. With the holidays coming up, I chose to make a pack of DIY transcendent oil formulas to impart to family, friends and neighbours. Eventually I will end up saving lots of money that could have been spent purchasing the unnatural products! Woot! Additionally, I also cherish the thought of giving friends and loved ones non-harmful gifts that they can use as toiletries or in their home.

Wanting to get started with basic oils?

Listed here you will find 18 of my main DIY Essential Oil formulas

Lavender Linen Spray

This can be a light splash that makes your clothing smell amazing and helps protect your health. After drying your clothes or sheets, spray or splash them with this Lavender Linen Spray for a wonderful and comforting aroma that will follow you all day. Since Lavender oil is gently, it is safe to use on your children's sheets before bed time. You could likewise utilize this as a relaxing body oil or fragrance (trade the refined water with light transporter oil like extracted coconut oil.)

What you'll need:

- 2 ounce dim glass splash bottle
- 1 teaspoon of witch hazel
- 15-20 drops of Lavender oil
- Nearly 2 ounces of refined water

Instructions:

Put the Lavender in your glass bottle. Add the witch hazel. Fill the rest of the bottle with refined water. Put on the splash top and shake bottle vigorously. Sprinkle on crisply washed pieces of clothing or on your mattress and sheets shortly before sleeping.

Cheats Spray

This flavourful oil mix smells like Christmas. I love this Cheats splash crucial oil formula and like to share it with my family and friends. It's easy to use, and I have one in my home and one in my diaper pack for travel.

You can use it to:

- Clean children's toys
- Clean public restroom seats
- Wipe down cutting boards
- Wash leafy foods
- Freshen gym bags
- Disinfect plane armrests and serving plates
- Spray inside the room to get rid of overwhelming smells

The uses of this spray are especially ceaseless. Also, it's super easy to make.

What you'll need:

- 2 oz. Darkish glass splash bottle
- 1 teaspoon common witch hazel
- 10-15 drops of youthful living Cheats oil
- Almost 2 oz. of refined water

Instructions:

For your perfect splash bottle, add 10-15 drops of your Cheats oil. Then add 1 tsp of witch hazel. Top up the bottle with refined water. . That is it! That is one of my favorite DIY crucial oil formulas!

Glossy Hair Serum

Who doesn't want thick, striking and magnificent hair? Generally because of stress, baby blues or age, our hair can start to thin, break or lose its radiance. I truly enjoy utilizing this DIY crucial oil formula to improve how my hair looks and smells.

What you'll need:

- 2 ounce darkish glass dropper bottle
- Close to 2 ounces of castor oil
- 10 drops of rosemary essential oil
- 5 drops of lavender crucial oil
- 5 drops of ylang premier oil

Instructions:

Pour 2 oz. of Castor Oil into your dropper bottle. Add the remaining oils. Put on dropper cover and shake bottle. Rub the mixture into your hair every morning. Leave it for up to 20 minutes then wash. It can be applied before bed, too! If you find the serum too oily, replace the castor oil with 2 oz. of refined water and 1 teaspoon of witch hazel.

All Intentions Salve

This is a top notch multi-purpose ointment that is great for your skin. Lemon and Melaleuca have various benefits including antibacterial. Lavender is a relaxing oil that is known for its effect on skin. I truly like having this ointment on hand. You can even use it as a hand moisturizer during the cold winter months.

What you'll need:

- 1 ounce glass moisturizer container
- 5 drops lemon oil
- 5 drops lavender oil
- 5 drops tea tree (melaleuca alternifolia) oil
- Nearly 2 oz. of uncooked coconut oil

Instructions:

Scoop 2 oz. of uncooked coconut oil directly into a little glass dish. Add the oils. Stir well with a steel fork or spoon. Scoop the mixture into your glass cream container and put the cover on. Store in a cool, dark place. Apply directly to skin as needed. This is a great one for moms!

Cozy Exfoliation Body Scrub

Is it accurate to say that our skin is our biggest organ? In order to care for it properly, we should be cleaning off the dead skin cells every day. Skin brushing is a great approach to this, especially if you combine it with a weekly body scrub. This extravagant peeling scrub will give your skin a beautiful shine!

What you'll need:

- eight ounce glass container
- White covers – not compulsory - for a unique look
- 4 oz. of uncooked olive oil
- 8 oz. of ocean / sea salt
- 5 drops each of lavender, frankincense and ylang

Instructions:

Measure your salt and empty directly into a large glass dish. Add the olive oil and mix well with a metallic spoon. Include your crucial oils and continue to blend your mixture. Gradually scoop into your glass container. Close firmly with a white cover and mark. Store in a cool, dark place. Scoop out a silver buck's-worth of scour and apply to body before showering. Repeat weekly. Your skin will thank you.

Pricey Exfoliation Facial Scrub

That is the same recipe above, however we use sugar instead of salt given that it's gentler and better for your face. I have three different oil combinations depending on your skin type.

What you'll need:
- 8 ounce glass container
- White lids – not obligatory but make for a unique look
- Half cup raw olive oil
- 1 cup raw sugar
- For normal skin: 5 drops each of Lavender, ylang and Frankincense
- For oily skin: 5 drops each of carrot seed oil, tea tree oil and frankincense
- For dry or older skin: 5 drops each of patchouli, geranium oil and frankincense
- For a special treat: 5 drops each of rose, jasmine and sacred frankincense oils

Instructions:
Measure your sugar and pour into a large glass bowl. Add your olive oil and blend well with a steel spoon. Add your crucial oils and continue to stir your mixture. Slowly scoop into your glass container. Close tightly with white lid and label. Store at room temperature in a dark place =. Scoop out a silver dollar's-worth of scrub and use weekly.

Muscle Love Bath Salts

These salts are perfect for athletes and people who need to ease their bodies after gruelling exercise or yard work.

What you'll need:

- eight ounce glass container
- White lids – not obligatory but it makes for a unique look
- 10 drops of panaway and/or aroma siez
- 5 drops of copiaba
- 1 cup of epsom salts

Instructions:

Put your Epsom salts into a large glass bowl. Add the crucial oils and blend well with a metallic spoon. Carefully pour into your eight ounce glass container and cover tightly with lid. Scoop out 1/4 to 1/2 cup and put into a warm bath when needed. The athlete in your life will be grateful!

Coffee Cellulite Scrub

That is the most unique of my DIY crucial oil recipes. Coffee is a recognized stimulant and may actually assist the body in breaking down fats deposits beneath the skin. Grapefruit and Cypress oils are also high-quality supporters of the lymph nodes. When mixed, this is a great scrub!

What you'll need:

- 8 ounce glass container
- White lids – not obligatory, choose your own color
- 10 drops of grapefruit oil
- 5 drops of cypress oil
- 1 cup natural espresso
- Half a cup of olive oil

Instructions:

Measure your coffee and pour into a large glass bowl. Add your olive oil and blend well with a metallic spoon. Add the oils and continue to stir your mixture. Slowly scoop into your glass container. Close tightly and label. Store in a cool, dark location. Scoop out a silver dollar's-worth amount of scrub and spread on your body before showering.

Balancing Fragrance Combination

Those with an exceptional sense of smell will love this perfume blend. I've given this to family members and friends many times. The combination of oils helps us feel bright and well. All of these oils are safe for children, pregnant mamas and breastfeeding mamas.

What you'll need:

- 1 darkish glass roll-on bottle
- ~ 1 TB extracted coconut oil
- 3 drops of grapefruit oil
- 2 drops of grankincense oil
- 1 drop of copiaba oil
- 1 drop of Bergamot oil

Instructions:

Add the oil drops to your roll-on bottle. Fill the remainder of your roll-on bottle with a mild carrier oil like extracted coconut oil. Close tightly. Preserve in a cool, dark location. Spread on pulse points as required.

Invigorating Cologne

Who says crucial oils are just for the ladies? Make your man a masculine roll on that will support his health and make him smell great. Balsam Fir provides a Christmas tree smell, and Cedar-wood has a musky scent that's superb for the guy in your life.

What you'll need:

- 1 dark glass roll-on bottle
- 1 TB abstracted coconut oil
- three drops of Balsam Fir oil
- three drops of Cedar wood oil

Instructions:

Add your oil drops to your roll-on bottle. Fill the rest of your roll-on bottle with a mild carrier oil like extracted coconut oil. Cover tightly. Store at room temperature in a dark location. Apply to pulse points as required.

Fresh Minty Shaving Cream

Do you know that the majority conventional shaving creams are stuffed with harsh chemicals and fragrances? I like this homemade concoction which leaves the skin feeling great, thanks to the shea and coconut oils, as well as invigorated as a result of the Peppermint oil. You can add any essential oil you'd like to vary up the scent.

What you'll need:
- 8 ounce glass container
- White lids – optional - it is up to your personal style
- 1/3 cup of shea butter
- 1/3 cup of coconut oil
- 3 TB uncooked olive oil
- 1 tsp castile soap
- 7-8 drops of peppermint oil

Instructions:
Put your shea spread and coconut oil in a twofold burner. Set on low heat and let the fats melt. Remove from the burner and empty your oils into a tumbler dish. Add your olive oil. Allow to cool and add your Castile soap and essential oil. Put in fridge for 60 minutes or until the mixture hardens. At that point, remove from the fridge and whip your mixture in a blender to form a whipped cream composition. Scoop into your glass container. Close tightly and store in a cool, dark place. Scoop out a silver buck's-worth of cream and apply before shaving.

Alleviating Shaving Gel

Men tend to prefer a gel rather than a cream, so I *invented* this blend for them to use. The aloe vera acts as the "gel" and leaves your skin smooth. Lemongrass and Grapefruit fragrance smell divine together and they encourage blood flow and the lymphatic system to work!

What you'll need:

- eight ounce dim glass pump bottle
- 3/4 cup aloe vera gel
- 1/4 cup olive oil
- 7 drops of lemongrass oil
- 7 drops of grapefruit oil

Instructions:

Using a funnel, pour the aloe vera gel into your glass. Add the olive oil and your key oils. Close your bottle with the pump cover and shake vigorously. Store in a cool, dim area. Whenever needed, spread onto the skin before shaving.

Arousing After Shave

This is also one of my top choices out of these DIY essential oil formulas for the reason that Orange + Sandalwood = Heaven! Each of these alleviating oils is perfect in this face ointment, not only because of the scent, but also because they hydrate the skin.

What you'll need:

- 8 ounce darkish glass pump bottle
- 1/2 cup aloe vera gel
- 1/2 cup witch hazel
- 2 TB jojoba oil
- 1 tsp vitamin E oil
- 10 drops orange oil
- 10 drops sandalwood oil

Instructions:

Using a funnel, pour the aloe vera gel into your jug. Then add the witch hazel, jojoba and vitamin E oils. Add the remaining ingredients. Close your compartment with the pump top and shake well. Store in a cool, dark area. Whenever needed, apply to the skin after shaving.

Mother's Boob and Stomach Rub

This rub is great for pregnant mothers. As our tummies and breasts expand during pregnancy and breastfeeding, this ointment will assist support the condition of your skin. Cocoa butter, shea butter, olive oil and vitamin E are commonly used in many skin ointments available on the market. These are all safe oils to use while pregnant and after birth.

What you'll need:
- eight ounce glass container
- White covers – or a color of your choosing
- 1/2 cup cocoa butter
- 1/2 cup shea butter
- 1/4 cup olive oil
- 1 TB of vitamin E
- 3-5 drops of geranium oil
- 3-5 drops of lavender oil

Instructions:
Put your cocoa and shea butter in a twofold burner on low heat and let the fats melt. Remove from the burner and place in a tumbler dish. Allow to cool then add your vitamin E, olive oil and other oils. Put in the fridge for 60 minutes or until it starts to harden. At that point, remove from the refrigerator and whip your mix in a blender until it forms a whipped cream surface. Scoop into your glass container. Close tightly and store in a cool, dark place. Spread on tummy and boobs daily as required.

Lethargic Spray

I like this mixture to help me sleep. It's a calming, soothing spray that blends certain oils with a specific sort of magnesium. Many of us lack this mineral as an after-effect of our drained soils or poor diet. Magnesium is additionally calming, so it's a double punch of serene goodness!

The secret to this formula is the magnesium oil, which acts as the "transporter oil." This transdermal wellspring of magnesium is gentler on the body than magnesium taken orally.

What you'll need:

- 2 ounce dim glass shower bottle
- Close to 2 oz. of old minerals magnesium oil
- 20 drops peace and calming (you may likewise utilize cedarwood, lavender, tangerine, or german / roman chamomile) oil

Instructions:

Fill your splash bottle with the magnesium oil. Add your crucial oils. Put on splash top and shake well. Apply 20 minutes before sleeping. Alternatively, open the bottle and breathe in the aroma as a calming agent.

Bubble Baths

There are things that can compare with the delight of a bubble bath. I can remember spending so much time surrounding by bubbles in my parent's bath, moulding Santa Claus beards and making towers and castles of bubbles. It is one of my favorite childhood memories.

So why have I been denying my children this experience?

Many bubble bath mixes available today have some generally horrendous ingredients... scents, parabens, even formaldehyde.
However, will that inconvenience stand in the way of a determined mother and her children's' bath time? Not in my home!

Make your own Bubble Bath

The best solution is to make your own bubble bath! That is top notch for the DIY-ers or individuals who wish to ensure their bubble bath is without poisons or toxins.
Recorded here are two or three formulas to try.

Soothing Salt Bubble Bath

The addition of magnesium-rich salt offers this bubble bath a calming and rejuvenating boost. First-class for calming youngsters and relieving growing pains!

- 1/2 cup epsom salt or magnesium flakes
- 1/8 cup himalayan pink salt (not obligatory)
- 1 cup liquid castile soap
- 1 tbsp. vegetable glycerin
- 30-50 drops essential Oils

Whisk all parts together. Drizzle underneath running water while filling the bath.

Moisturizing Honey Bubble Bath

The honey and almond oil in this recipe are ideal for moisturizing dry skin or for kids with eczema.

- 1 cup sweet almond oil
- 1/2 cup honey
- 3/4 cup liquid castile soap
- 30-50 drops of crucial oils (Lavender works well)

Whisk all parts together. Drizzle underneath running water while filling the bathtub.

Super Bubble Bath

The egg white in this recipe helps the bubbles preserve their form longer.

- 1 cup liquid castile cleaning soap
- 1 egg white
- 30-50 drops essential oils

Whisk all ingredients together. Drizzle underneath running water while filling the bath. For extra foaming vigour, add a bit of water and mix with a hand mixer to make more foam before filling the bath.

You can also add 1 cup of water to stretch this recipe and make it last longer. It will not be as bubbly, however it will save money.

Why we restrict our child's baths

Bubble baths are extremely good, however you should nonetheless restrict them to about once per week in your household.

Our skin hosts good bacteria that shouldn't be washed away too often. That's why skin-to-skin touching is so important to new-borns who're establishing their micro biome.

The "hygiene speculation" states that too few exposures to micro-organisms and pathogens in early childhood may have a negative impact on proper immune development. Research has determined that bathing too often may lead to eczema, bronchial asthma, leukaemia and even diabetes.

Washing away the normal oils (sebum) on our skin too often can cause dry skin or could cause the skin to enter sebum overdrive which leads to oily skin.

Also, the normal oils on our skin support absorption of Vitamin D from the sun. Your skin can take up to 48 hours to entirely absorb vitamin D via the skin, so washing too frequently could affect healthy Vitamin D levels.

A bit of a downer about bubble baths, right? But, in moderation, bubble baths can be healthy and super fun.

Mommy likes a good bubble bath too!

You're on no account too old to revel in your own bubble bath! I like to add a couple of drops of Lavender, Chamomile Peace & Calming or Stress Away crucial oil to my baths for additional therapeutic relaxation.

How about you?

Do your children take bubble baths? What bubble bath do you use?

Conclusion

Scientists are continually watching for new and improved approaches to the cleansing products we use in our everyday lives. Nevertheless, the answer lies not in chemistry but in nature. Why artificially produce chemical-heavy products when it's possible to create them from natural substances that aren't only perfectly able to do the job, but are also beneficial to the human body?

Previously we examined the vitality of essential oils, especially their antitoxin properties. Crucial oils are great for distinctive areas of soothing, cleansing, freshening, etc., and I have shown you probably the easiest methods in which you are able to create absolutely natural, yet nonetheless robust, products at home.

In all honestly, there is no better alternative than creating homemade products with the use of essential oils.